THE CHOICE

MEDICINE VS. NURSING

Which field is right for you?

Shirie Leng RN, MSN, MD

INTRODUCTION

Since I started blogging about healthcare and health policy a few years ago, by far the most common questions I get are from students trying to decide between a career in nursing and a career in medicine. Here are quotes from some of my readers:

I graduated from college with a BA in biochemistry, hoping to pursue medical school after taking a gap year. Now, I'm torn between MD and NP (which I would enter [via an]accelerated bsn/ msn program). I love the science and extensive medical training that comes with being an MD, but I am also worried about the debt, stress, and years ahead before I can start to practice independently. On the other hand, being an NP, I would finish school sooner, with less debt, and will be a mid-level practitioner that could still diagnose and treat patients.

I'm 25 years old and would love to have children at some point but my husband doesn't think it's feasible right now or even after getting my MD. (He is 30 and in DPT school currently) so our career choices are both very demanding and time isn't really on our side in my opinion). My question is how did you manage your educational goals while simultaneously raising 3 children?

I have done a semester of an RN program but I'm starting to have an identity crisis. If I worked harder in the past, I would have been going to medical school today. I do like personally handing PO medications. On the other hand, I least like inflicting pain with injections. I like taking care of patients and tending to their needs, but I crave the knowledge that doctors have.

When I was in college I was premed, but had doubts of getting into a program. I thought NP was the closest next best and I pursued it and got into an excellent program. Now seeing in reality what NP, RN, CRNA, MDs do, I'm still left with doubt. Some places accept the role of an NP well and others don't. Many clinics I have worked with have MD/NP on the same playing field but I have not seen that in most hospitals. I am 25, single, no children, and no plans for until much much later, and I find myself pondering going to medical school. I have been studying for my MCAT... but fearful that I will be 30, in residency and wishing I was an NP.

Having applied to both nursing and medical school, how was the process different for you? If you were to do it over again, would you have gone the NP/CRNA route? As a nurse, would it be easier to have a work/lifestyle balance than an MD?

Hi! I'm a sophomore in college and I saw that you said you are a doctor and a nurse. How does that work and is it looked down upon sometimes? I've recently been thinking of majoring in nursing instead of going to medical school. And I honestly don't know what I want to do... I was actually kind of wanting to be a nurse and a doctor, but I was advised not to do so and that it doesn't look good to say that when applying to either nursing school or medical school.

I'm trying to decide between going to an accelerated NP program... or doing premed requirements and going the MD route. I am 31! I worry I'm to old to start med school. I'm also worried about going to med school when I am around the age of wanting to start a family etc.

I am supposed to start an accelerated second-degree BSN/MSN program in two weeks, at the age of 27. I love the idea of having flexibility all along my career path, and the academics and structure of these programs seem so manageable to me. However, I have a strong desire to know the ins-and-outs of medicine and understand the pathophysiology/pharmacology at least as well as anyone else in my field. When I speak to physicians, they say that the NPs and PAs never quite reach the same level of understanding as physicians. This gives me great pause.

If any of these writers' words sound familiar, this is the book for you!

CHAPTER 1

WHY WE CHOOSE BADLY

Barry Schwartz, in his book *The Paradox of Choice*, cogently expresses the importance of understanding how we choose:

With many decisions, the consequences of error may be trivial - a small price to pay for the wealth of choices available to us. But with some, the consequences of error may be quite severe. We may make bad investments because we are not well informed enough about the tax consequences of investing in the various possibilities. We may choose the wrong health plan because we don't have time to read all the fine print. We may go to the wrong school, choose the wrong courses, embark on the wrong career, all because of the way in which the options were presented to us. As we find more and more important decisions on our plates, we may be forced to make many of those decisions with inadequate reflection. And in these cases, the stakes can be high.

There is no better story to illustrate the perils of decision-making than my own.

As a kid I had always thought I would become a nurse. It is unclear from whence this idea came. My grandmother was a nurse, or so I was told as she quit when she married my grandfather. (A doctor, of course. This was the 1920s after all.) I knew some nurses. I had read the wonderful series of books by Helen Wells about a nurse named Cherry Ames. Cherry Ames, department store nurse! Cherry Ames, dude ranch nurse! Never mind that I was a band camp book nerd who almost failed out of algebra several times and had never set foot in a chemistry lab. I wasn't at all worried about the fact that I had no idea what nursing was all about.

I also played the violin. Apparently I played with enough skill to be considered at least mildly talented. The adults around me encouraged me to major in music, although I was pretty sure I would never be good enough to be a professional. In my own narrative I would like to say that my mom, a wonderful pianist, really wanted me to, although I have no idea if this was true. But I was flattered, and I was obedient. So I went to music school.

After music school, terrified I wasn't good enough to be a professional violinist, terrified of auditions, and without a job, I babysat around New York City until I landed on the idea, once again, of nursing. The main attractions at that point, I'm afraid, were that nursing wasn't music, there was no audition, and it paid better than babysitting.

So I went to Yale. This made my parents happy and took me off the hook from having to deal with real life and student loans. I did the Non-nurse College Graduate Program, as it was then called, a three-year program in which you are RN-eligible at 2 years and complete a Master's degree in the final year. It's a wonderful program with great nurse-scholars and fantastic students.

Of course, once I got a job as a nurse, I didn't like it. It was hard work. My feet hurt all the time. Patients were always asking for things. That's what I told myself, although in truth nursing was never going to be a good fit for me. My decision-making process had been non-existent.

Being stubborn and only 25, I decided what I really needed to do was to be a doctor. It didn't look too hard. I had friends who were doctors. I worked with doctors. It wasn't nursing. That was pretty much the sum of my thought process. I knew what I was getting into.

Dear reader, I had no idea.

HOW WE CHOOSE

An extensive amount of data now exists in the science of choice. Social researchers such as David Kahneman and Dan Ariely have conducted numerous experiments which suggest a number of ways in which humans are led astray when making choices. An understanding some of these pitfalls is critical as you embark on the process of deciding between medicine and nursing. They are problems I should have understood much earlier than I did. I present here just a few. A list of recommended books can be found at the end of the chapter

Prospect Theory

Prospect theory is one of the most well known explanations of how we evaluate options and make decisions. Gaining and losing are not weighted equally in our minds. Gaining something makes us happier only to a certain point, and then the effect of gain lessens. By contrast, losing something generates negative feelings to a far greater degree than gaining something creates positive feelings. The dividing line between what is gain and what is loss, and our tolerance for both, is different for every person and every situation.

Loss is a more powerful motivator than gain. This is one of the most potent instincts humans have. We are wired to react much more negatively to having lost something than to never having gained it. This concept is particularly important for the purposes of this book, because the loss of choice that results from having *made* a choice can be very painful. If I decide to have a child, let's say, the loss of the *possibility* of going out to dinner or a movie whenever I want is painful, even if I never choose to go to the movies or dinner. The loss of the option is what hurts. If I decide to marry X, I've closed the door on a potential better fit in an unknown Y - even if I never meet Y.

If you decide definitively on medicine you might not feel that you have gained the commitment to a great career but that you've lost the possibility of family, leisure, and care-free weekends. Even if you don't have a family yet, and even if your assumptions about the life-style of doctors are wrong. If you decide to major in nursing as an undergraduate, rather than feeling that you've gained a steady, fulfilling, and well-paid career you might feel you've lost the possibility of becoming a doctor. Even if you don't really want to be a doctor.

Beware of "keeping your options open".

Having a whole bunch of options is not necessarily a good thing. Having loss as a motivator is actually a luxury. If you had no choice, you'd not experience a loss of options. Too many choices tends to paralyze people. Let's take a look at a quote from one of my readers.

...if you feel passionate about or like multiple fields equally (i.e anesthesiology, cardiology, heme/onc) and both nursing and medicine seem to fit well with multiple specialties more or less equally, how would you decide?

This poor student is not only trying to decide between medicine and nursing, but about what specialty to choose within each! It turns out that a large array of options can discourage people from actually deciding because it increases the effort involved in making the choice. Too many choices tends to paralyze people. One way people try to get around this is to get someone else to make the decision for them. For example, when my husband decides to buy something, he likes to comparison shop online. This process often takes weeks because there are so many options. Eventually he will throw up his hands and say "whatever you think, honey".

Another way people compensate when confronted with too much choice is they decide not to decide by choosing the option that closes the least amount of doors (prospect theory). Here is another example of a reader questioning his decisions:

As I am in school completing my pre-requisites for the nursing program, I have a strong desire to become a physician, specifically a DO. I am thinking about becoming a doctor maybe after I work a few years as an RN and after I pursue my music career endeavors.

Making the choice to do nursing "while I decide if I want to be a doctor" is not really a choice at all. It does a disservice to the field of professional nursing for one thing. Nursing is not "medicine lite" as we will see in subsequent chapters. The quote demonstrates this student's desperate attempt to avoid the loss of options. Paradoxically, this choice which is not a choice will actually diminish the student's enjoyment of the real choice he finally makes. His commitment to and enjoyment of the field he chooses will be diminished as he looks over the fence at the roads not taken. Barry Schwartz says that "A large array of options may diminish the attractiveness of what people *actually* choose, the reason being that thinking about the attractions of some of the unchosen options detracts from the pleasure derived from the chosen one."

Availability Heuristic

This is a term Daniel Kahneman, in his book *Thinking, Fast and Slow*, and his colleague Amos Tversky use to refer to our tendency to choose what is most prominent in our minds. An heuristic is a rule of thumb or mental shortcut. When faced with a choice some types of information will have more weight than other types. This is partly why after a terrorist attack in one country people in a completely different part of the world will rate terrorism higher on their list of fears than, say, driving their cars, even though the chance of being directly affected by a terrorist attack is very small compared to the chance of being in an auto accident.

Another example of the availability heuristic has to do with where our information comes from. If I go to a nursing website like allnurses.com I will get a lot of information about what nurses think about various issues, what they feel about their work, and an overall general impression of nursing as a profession. This view of nursing, although it is gathered from hundreds of sources, will have much less of an impact on my decision to become a nurse than colorful anecdotes or horror stories told to me by my nursing friends yesterday at lunch.

Imprinting

The converse does not turn out to be true, however. If I decide to be a nurse and commit to that decision *before* someone tells me something negative about nursing, I'm much less likely to listen to them. If something looks like what you've already decided it is, you will look for evidence to back up your decision instead of being open to all possibilities. We tend to make decisions that cohere with past decisions and not necessarily with our current preferences. This was one of my own major errors. Having made a decision, I was no longer interested in any evidence that my decision was wrong.

When we choose one thing and go with it forever, assuming that choice continues to be the right one without ever thinking it through again, we are imprinting. It happens in the mother-child bond. It is very similar to what in medicine we would call premature closure. Premature closure occurs when, say, an overweight middle-aged man presents with chest pain and the doctor decides immediately that it the man is suffering from a heart attack. He then looks for evidence to back up his diagnosis, ignoring or discounting opposing evidence that suggests it is esophageal reflux disease that is causing the patient's discomfort. Medical school has imprinted the image of a typical patient presenting with a heart attack, and the doctor goes with it.

Comparison

Humans have an innate habit of comparing things. It starts very young, when 3-year-olds worry about who has the most crayons and 5-year-olds compare Christmas presents. We also see things within a certain context, comparing items within the milieu of what we have recently experienced. What we see tends to change depending on what things are next to each other or what thing we've seen most recently. My Honda Civic looks great in the parking lot next to that rusted Sirocco but like a piece of junk next to the Audi A8 on the other side. Being a nurse looks great compared to your high school friend who works at Starbucks but maybe not so great when measured against another friend who pilots fighter planes.

Bias

What society leads us to believe has a very important impact on what we choose. Our own biases and assumptions blind us to possibilities. Similarly, what other people think tends to weigh heavily on us. We compare what we've become with what others think we should have become or become what we think will get the most people to think well of us. The problem here, of course, is that everyone sees the world through their own eyes and their thoughts and judgements are based in whatever biases they have. When somebody says "You're so smart, you should go to medical school!" they are imposing a set of biases and assumptions on your decision. That you believe it when someone tells you this has to do not only with your own biases but your tendency to want to be thought well of.

Framing

Our decisions can also be influenced by the way information is presented, not only in context or point of view but visually as well. Kahneman and Tversky call the presentation of the same option in different ways "framing". If you presented the pros and cons of nursing on nice paper with colors and attractive font, while presenting medicine on copy paper in black and white Helvetic, I'd be more likely to choose nursing. Works in menus and book covers too.

The Crystal Ball Effect

Knowing what you want is influenced by the relationships you have with the present, future, and past. Knowing what you want means being able to anticipate *in the now* how you will feel *in the future* if you choose different options *based on your experience in the past*. Food shopping is the classic example of this. When you go to the store you buy a food now that you predict you will like when you eat it later because you've had the same or a similar food in the past. Kent Greenfield, in his book *The Myth of Choice* puts it this way:

Our ability to make anything close to a good decision in the present depends not only on our judgements about what we want, think, and feel right now but on our memories of what we wanted, thought, and felt in past and our predictions about what we will want, think, and feel in the future.(Pg 66)

This is unfortunate because, while it's easy to predict the future when it comes to lunch, it is a bit different when we are trying to predict how we will feel about a decision that will affect us ten years from now. Not only is it hard to tell how we will feel about something we've never done, but ten years from now the goals we have might change completely.

Frankly, it seems like in order to know what you want you have to *know yourself.* In chapter 2 we'll look at some ways to accomplish this.

Recommended reading:

Ariely, Dan. *Predictably Irrational.* Harper Perennial, New York, 2009.

Duhigg, Charles. *The Power of Habit.* Random House, New York, 2012.

Greenfield, Kent. *The Myth of Choice.* Yale University Press, New Haven, CT, 2012.

Iyengar, Sheena. *The Art of Choosing.* Twelve, Grand Central Publishing, New York, 2010.

Kahneman, Daniel. *Thinking, Fast and Slow.* Farrah, Straus and Giroux, New York, 2011,

Lehrer, Jonah. *How We Decide.* Houghton Mifflin, New York, 2009.

Schwartz, Barry. *The Paradox of Choice.* Harper Perennial, New York, 2005.

CHAPTER 2

WHAT DO YOU WANT?

Now that you know some of the ways our thinking leads us to poor decisions, let's look at Barry Schwartz's six steps to better decision-making:

1. Figure out what your goals are.
2. Evaluate how important each goal is.
3. Gather all your options.
4. Evaluate how likely each option is to fulfill each goal.
5. Pick a winning option.
6. Re-evaluate.

These steps sound simple enough. You probably think you've already been through them several times. Here's the problem. Step number 1 can take you your whole life to answer, because step number 1 forces you to ask the following question: *What do you want?*

Let's take a simple example. You go to the library. Your goal is to find a book to read that you will like. The book should be interesting and have historical figures and political intrigue. The decision to go to the library for your book is based on prior experience with other sources of books, such as bookstores, your experience with the particularly library you go to, and an evaluation of your current book situation, that is, your overburdened bookshelves. Once in the library, you have to make more choices. If you think you want fiction you can go to the new fiction section, or to the stacks with the older publications. But wait, maybe you don't want fiction. The last book of fiction you read was historical fiction and you thought it was too sappy and overly romantic. Your most important goal is to avoid sappy. So, surveying your options, you decide to go to the biography section. You have no experience with biography, but you liked History 101 in college and it must be better than your recent experiences with fiction, plus there are bound to be historical figures, also one of your goals. You go with a book about Abraham Lincoln because you saw the movie last week and there was plenty of interesting history and political intrigue in it. You leave the library hoping you made a good choice, but only upon reading the book will you know if the choice was correct or not.

It sounds silly, but we go through this process all the time with things that don't matter very much. You're hungry. Your goal is food that is salty, not sweet, with a little carbohydrate and a lot of protein. You look in the fridge, evaluate how close the things in it are to your food goals, pick something, and decide if you like it. The problem is that when the stakes are higher, the process tends to get stuck, and it often goes off the rails at step number 1.

There are places to go for help but, as we will see, they are not perfect.

PERSONALITY TESTING

Humans love tests. Not the mid-term kind, necessarily, but the kind that purport to reveal something about ourselves to us. Anyone who has ever taken the "Cosmo Quiz" or participated in the "What kind of (fill in the blank) are you?" quizzes on Facebook knows how tempting these things can be. If only a small number of questions about what we like or what we might do in a given situation could answer all our questions about life and love!

The world of psychology has come up with its own, more complete and better tested versions of the Cosmo Quiz. The most famous of these is the Myers-Briggs test.

The Myers-Briggs Type Indicator (MBTI)

The MBTI was developed by Katharine Cook Briggs and her daughter Isabel Briggs Myers. Believe it or not, the idea originated because Katharine was trying to decide if a man named Clarence was good enough to marry Isabel. Her research led her to Carl Jung, the famous Swiss psychiatrist, who had published a book called *Psychological Types* in 1923. He proposed that people are innately different in the way they see the world, take in information, and make decisions. Myers-Briggs testing results in the sorting of normal people into 16 types. Everyone, according to Isabel Myers, has a personality that can be characterized by questions intended to get at your preferences in four general categories and, although all of these functions exist in all of us, one feature of each scale is usually dominant.

1. Favorite world: Do you prefer to focus on the outer world (Extraversion) or on your own inner world (Introversion)?
2. Information: Do you prefer to focus on the basic information you take in (Sensing) or do you prefer to interpret and add meaning (Intuition)?
3. Decisions: When making decisions, do you prefer to first look at logic and consistency (Thinking) or first look at the people and special circumstances (Feeling)?

4.Structure: In dealing with the outside world, do you prefer to get things decided (Judging) or do you prefer to stay open to new information and options (Perceiving)?

Lucky for us in terms of the subject matter of this book, early forms of the MBTI were tested, beginning in 1951, on medical students. With 5,355 medical students (men) from 45 medical colleges signed up, the goal was to determine which types might end up more content in the medical profession and which types would end up choosing certain medical specialties. The results were presented by Isabel Myers at the American Psychological Association conference in 1964.

Most medical students were identified as carrying the personality type INFP, meaning that they looked at the world in ways that indicated preferences for Introversion, Intuition, Feeling, and Perceiving. What does this mean? For that we turn to the Myers-Briggs Foundation. According to the foundation's website, here's the definition of an INFP:

Idealistic, loyal to their values and to people who are important to them. Want an external life that is congruent with their values. Curious, quick to see possibilities, can be catalysts for implementing ideas. Seek to understand people and to help them fulfill their potential. Adaptable, flexible, and accepting unless a value is threatened.

But wait! The study also determined the most typical personality type seen in surgeons: ESTP.

Flexible and tolerant, they take a pragmatic approach focused on immediate results. Theories and conceptual explanations bore them - they want to act energetically to solve the problem. Focus on the here-and-now, spontaneous, enjoy each moment that they can be active with others. Enjoy material comforts and style. Learn best through doing.

What happened? Did medical students change their personality between the first day and the last day of medical school? Well yes, in a way. Studies have shown that personality can change over time due to life-changing experiences - either traumatic or joyful - as well as simple growth and maturation. Some have found that personality traits do indeed change but usually in the direction of traits becoming more pronounced.

Whatever the reason, the real takeaway here is that determining your personality type does not seem to be terribly helpful in career decision-making when it comes to nursing and medicine. Your INFP internal medicine doctor could just as easily be a pediatric nurse. The ESTP could be an emergency room nurse just as well as a trauma surgeon.

It turns out you find all MBTI personality types in virtually all specialties in both nursing and medicine. This is because, for the nurse or the doctor, personality informs and colors *how* the individual will practice much more than it determines *what* the person will practice.

The DiSC Personal Profile System

There are a ton of personality tests out there, but let's take a look at one that does not purport to tell you what you might want to do with your life, but rather what your personality says about how you will do anything you choose. The DiSC, developed by Dr. Robert Rohm, identifies four dimensions of behavior: dominance (D), influence (i), steadiness (S) and conscientiousness (C).

A person with a dominant personal style likes action, results, fast-moving work, and being in charge - - your garden variety trauma surgeon or ER nurse. A person with predominantly i characteristics is better with people and relationships, such as anyone in pediatrics or psychiatry, while a steady personality is loyal, calm, and dependable, your good old anesthesiologist or nurse anesthetist. A conscientious person likes accuracy, standards, detail, and analytics, a perfect fit for nursing administration.

Sounds like this personality test might be appropriate. Except…wouldn't it be great to have a loyal, calm, and dependable trauma surgeon? Of course! Would patients love to have an ER nurse who is good with people? Absolutely! And you certainly would not say no to a nurse anesthetist who likes accuracy and detail.

Self-Evaluation

Personality testing is really just a standardized way to evaluate yourself and your preferences. Howard Figler of *The Complete Job-Search Handbook* and Richard Nelson Bolles of the famous *What Color is your Parachute?* don't depend much on personality metrics. Howard Figler explains that:

People are only too willing to submit themselves to someone who will 'tell me who I am and what I should do with my life.' People want to discover their futures, and they believe that anyone except themselves can tell them about it. Test results imply that the high scores are where the person is more likely to be satisfied and successful. However, predictive validity studies seldom appear in test manuals, and I know of no studies that have ever shown significant prediction of career outcomes.

Mr. Figler has found that clients tend to lean heavily on such testing, and many career counselors do too, the client because he thinks the test has the power to predict his future and the counselor because it seems like a good place to start.

Like Mr. Figler, Richard Bolles rejects multiple choice tests in favor of questions intended to get at what kind of person a client is. He uses open-ended questions such as these:

1. What do you know? What are your favorite fields of knowledge?
2. What kinds of people do you like to hang out with and work with?
3. What can you do? What are your favorite skills?
4. What are your ideal working conditions?
5. What is your preferred level of responsibility?

6. What is your favorite geographical location?
7. What are your goals, or sense of mission and purpose?

      The answers to these questions require you to understand who you are and what you want. No one can really do that for you, but sometimes it helps to have someone else do the asking. The key thing to make sure of, when you are trying to answer these and many other questions about yourself, is to *be honest* with yourself. If you know, for sure, that you really hate being awakened in the middle of the night, fine. Own it. Don't try to hedge and pretend that you won't mind it when lives are at stake. You will totally mind. If all your friends are bookish types who like classical music, don't pretend to yourself that you'll be fine hanging out in the OR all day with people who talk sports and listen to Jay Z.

      The hardest of Bolles's questions to answer, of course, is number 7, which is why it is Schwarz's *first* question. You have to be specific. The goal I hear most often is "I want to help people." Great. The waitress at my local diner helps people. So does my cleaning lady. Even a lawyer might help the occasional soul. Same thing with "I want to make a difference." Believe me, my babysitter makes more difference in my life than anyone I've ever met.

Know what you want.

Recommended Reading:

Bolles, Richard N. *What Color is Your Parachute?*. 2014 ed. Ten Speed Press, New York.

Figler, Howard and Bolles, Richard N. *The Career Counselor's Handbook.* 2nd ed. Ten Speed Press, Berkley, 2007.

Lore, Nicholas. *The Pathfinder.* 2nd ed. Touchstone, Simon and Schuster, New York, 2011.

For more information on personality testing:

Janda, Louis. *The Psychologists Book of Personality Tests.* John Wiley & Sons, Hoboken, NJ, 2001.

Quenk, Naomi. *Essentials of Myers-Briggs Type Indicator Assessment.* 2nd ed. John Wiley & Sons, Hoboken, NJ, 2009.

Rohm, Robert. *Positive Personality Profiles.* 11th ed. Personality Insights, Inc, Atlanta, GA, 2000.

CHAPTER 3

FALSE ASSUMPTIONS

If, after chapters 1 and 2, you have made progress on Schwartz decision-making steps 1 and 2, you are ready to move on to step 3: gather options. Since you are reading this book I'll assume you've gathered two basic options: nursing or medicine. These are not, in fact, your only options, by the way. Don't lock yourself in. That said, if you really know something in the health sciences is right for you, you have to deal with step 4: evaluating each option. You can't do that unless you have an in-depth, unbiased, and accurate knowledge of what each field involves.

Let's do a little experiment. Let's make a pro and con list for nursing as it might have appeared when I was making the choice to go to nursing school. Knowing nothing about nursing except that Cherry Ames wore cute clothes and was perpetually young, here's my list:

PRO	CON
It gives me a goal	none
Makes my parents happy	none
Steady paycheck	none
Job security	none
That cap…	Wait, nurses don't wear caps anymore?
Meet cute doctors	none

What a horrible list! I was so focused on what I thought nursing could do for me, based on nothing but stereotypes, that I was blinded to any potential problems with my decision.

Now fast forward to my decision to go into medicine. Here's what my list might have looked like:

PRO	CON
Respect and authority	Long educational road
Better pay	Expensive education
Makes me look smarter	none
Get to have doctors as colleagues	none
Don't have to be a nurse anymore	none

Same horrible list, same problems.

Stereotypes

Now, let's look at what a comparison list of nursing and medicine might look like if you were using stereotypes from media sources, books, TV, and movies.

DOCTOR	NURSE
Give all the orders	Has to do whatever the doctor says
Wear the white coats, ties, and nice shoes. Or sexy scrubs with mask hanging down.	Wear ill-fitting cotton clothing, preferably with flowers or teddy bears on them
Good-looking	Good-looking, or really unattractive
Dates and/or sleeps with nurses (if male)	Wants to date and/or sleep with doctors (either sex)
Is kind of a b#@$% (if female)	Are the nice ones, give hugs and look sympathetic. Unless looking outraged.
Have lots of money, drive nice cars	Toyota, preferably hybrid. Less money
Don't get their hands dirty. Unless operating, and then only a teeny bit of blood.	Bring drinks

These lists are meant to be funny, but they also underscore how little accurate information many of us have about what we are choosing. These lists are based on *expectations* rather than reality. Do not underestimate the influence expectations and stereotyping have on decision-making.

Comparison

We don't choose in isolation. We make comparisons. We focus on the perceived relative value of one thing over another. Let's look at one more chart, a little more serious. This one provides a side-by-side comparison that might be written by someone who is trying to make a good decision but is still mired in stereotype.

DOCTOR	NURSE
It takes a long time to become a doctor.	Nursing has a much shorter educational course than medicine.
It costs a lot to become a doctor	Nursing school is cheaper than medical school.
Doctors don't do a lot of direct patient care.	Nurses do most of the actual care of a patient.
Doctors give orders and make all the decisions.	Nurses do what the doctors say.
Doctors are well-respected.	Nurses are not well-respected.
Doctors have a lot of responsibility.	Nurses don't have as much responsibility as doctors.
Doctors work more hours.	Nurses don't work as many hours.
Doctors can wear nice clothes unless they are operating.	Nurses wear scrubs.

This list doesn't work because the assumptions are wrong. But what if we did a little more research and tried to make a more informed comparison? The US Department of Labor, in its Employment and Training Administration arm, has an Occupational Information Network, or O*Net. O*Net online has a set of what it calls Summary Reports, that list the tasks, knowledge base, work styles, values, abilities, and interests for a wide variety of jobs. I looked up the Summary Report for Registered Nurse and compared it to one for General Internist.

GENERAL INTERNIST	REGISTERED NURSE
treat	maintain
prescribe	administer
explain	record
manage	monitor
analyze	coordinate
advise	prepare

Well, this is a load of baloney. This chart makes it look like the Internist decides what's to be done and the nurse stands around and takes notes! The truth, as we will discover, is that both doctors and nurses do all these things in one way or another. All these comparisons are terrible, because the two fields are, at their core, *completely different.*

CHAPTER 4

WHAT IS NURSING?

Now that we know how useless it is to compare medicine and nursing as career choices, how our decision-making runs off the rails, and how inaccurate a lot of our information is, let's examine these two different fields in detail. I'm going to start with the story of one woman who had the choice to go to medical school and chose nursing instead.

Margaret's Story

Margaret Moss had always known she was going to be a doctor. She grew up on the grounds of a Veteran's Administration hospital where her father was a doctor and her mother a nurse. She had memorized every bone in the body by the time she was in sixth grade. As soon as she could she got a job making pocket money as a nurse's aide. She majored in Biology at the University of North Dakota and did all her pre-med courses. She took the MCAT and did very well, applied to medical school and got wait-listed for the University of North Dakota Medical School. While she waited, she went to the National Cancer Institute, working in one of their basic science labs.

Spending all that time in the lab, she began to wonder if she was on the right track. She was still working as a nurse's aide sporadically. What she decided was this: "I really like people. I like taking care of people. So while I was [in the lab waiting for medical school to start] I thought I would try nursing."

She got her two-year nursing diploma (ADN). She began working as a staff nurse at the VA and loved it. From that point on, nursing has always made sense for her.

After deciding that nursing was the right choice for her, she went to work for Indian Health Services. Margaret herself is Native American. She ended up working as a nurse at the Santa Fe Hospital in New Mexico. "It was fantastic," she says. "I loved every minute of it." As an Indian from the plains of the Dakotas, she found the people and culture of the Pueblo Indians different and fascinating. As someone who was instantly accepted as Indian by the patients she cared for, she became a supervisor at the Santa Fe hospital and a patient education specialist.

Margaret began to notice that the the elderly Pueblo Indians never sought medical care in an Anglo or Hispanic health facility. Since at the time there weren't any Indian facilities, the patients would simply die at home. She decided to create a culturally-specific Indian elder daycare facility. She wanted to write up a business plan but didn't know anything about business. So she went and got a Master's degree in Administration Management. While working on implementing her ideas in Rio Rancho, New Mexico, she started to work on a doctorate in gerontology. While obtaining a PhD in gerontology, she eventually got a grant from the National Institute of Aging to do an ethnography study with the Indians of the Sunni Pueblo, who are one of the most culturally traditional Indian tribes in existence today.

What she found was stunning. In this traditional culture the elderly firmly believe in the dictates of the priest or medicine man. They believe that the things the priest decreed that must be done *must be done.* These dictates include things like going out in the morning at dawn on certain days in which the ancestors were close by, touching the earth and making a plate of food which they share with the ancestors, and fasting with the lunar calendar and other times the priest calls for it. The elders believe that if they don't do these things they bring evil and death upon their families, the pueblo, and the world at large. Traditional hospitals won't or can't accommodate these sorts of requirements. The Indians had learned this, so they just didn't go to hospitals or clinics at all.

Dr. Moss, as she now was called, having finished her PhD, tried to create a nursing home for these elderly Indians in which accommodations could be made for these traditional and religious rituals. However, she encountered legal problems, having to do with a state moratorium on building new nursing homes. While navigating state and federal government agencies for waivers, she realized that the Indians didn't know US law, that no one was helping them, and that no one could put the pieces together.

So, Margaret being Margaret, she went to law school. She went to work in health policy in Washington DC as a Robert Wood Johnson health policy fellow, and is now on the faculty of the Yale University School of Nursing. Here is what she says about her career:

If I had never been a nurse [in the Indian Health Service] I probably would have never put two and two and two together. State laws don't jibe with the things I learned. I feel bottom line my call was nursing. I couldn't fight the calling. I couldn't have had the career I've had if I had become a doctor. I'm a nurse.

History of Nursing

The act of nursing, that is the act of taking care of someone who is sick, has, of course, been around forever. Anyone who looks after a vomiting child, a feverish husband, or an injured dog is nursing. Professional nursing, in which people get paid to nurse others, has been around since the Roman Empire. What we now think of as the profession of nursing, encompassing theory, research, education, and regulation, originated in the 1860s with Florence Nightingale. As the founder of modern nursing Ms. Nightingale is a good person to turn to as we start our discussion of what nursing is and what nurses do. In an 1859 publication entitled *Notes on Nursing: What It Is and What It Is Not* she says the following:

I use the word nursing for want of a better. It has been limited to signify little more than the administration of medicines and the application of poultices. It ought to signify the proper use of fresh air, light, warmth, cleanliness. quiet and the proper selection and administration of diet - all at the least expense of vital power to the patient.

In other words, professional nursing is much more than carrying out the orders of doctors. The nurse's area of expertise lies in setting up the environment in such a way as to promote what Nightingale calls the "reparative process".

Nursing Philosophy and Theory

Ms. Nightingale's ideas coalesced into a nursing philosophy, that in turn gave rise to the modern construction of nursing theory.

The underlying concept here is that as a profession nursing has a body of knowledge that is distinct from any other profession. Beth Perry Black, in the 7th edition of *Professional Nursing: concepts and challenges*, says this:

Nursing as a profession has a distinct theoretical orientation to practice. This means that the practice of nursing is based on a specific body of knowledge that is built on theory. This body of knowledge shapes and is shaped by how nurses see the world.

Here are some examples of how Nightingale and those that followed her formulated their theories, taken from Beth Perry Black:

Florence Nightingale

When confronted with a patient, Ms. Nightingale asks, "What needs to be adjusted in this environment to protect the patient and promote healing?"

Virginia Henderson

When confronted with a patient, Ms. Henderson asks, "What can I help this patient do that he would do for himself if he could?"

Jean Watson

When confronted with a patient, Ms. Watson asks, "How can I create an environment of trust, understanding, and openness so that the patient and I can work together in meeting his or her needs?"

Dorthea Orem

When confronted with a patient, Ms. Orem asks, "What deficits does this patient have in providing his or her own self-care?"

Imogene King

When confronted with a patient, Ms. King asks, "What goals can we set together to restore the patient to heart?"

Callista Roy

When confronted with a patient, Ms. Roy asks, "How can I modify this patient's environment to facilitate his or her adaptation?"

You get the general idea. Nursing seeks to help people with activities until they regain the ability to do those activities for themselves, and to create an environment that makes reclaiming these abilities possible.

Let me try to explain how nursing theory works as an example. I'm going to use the Roper-Logan-Tierney "Activities of Living" model. This theory is based the work of Virginia Henderson, and is most used these days in the UK. Today we usually abbreviate activities of daily living to ADL. Here are the activities of daily living (ADLs) that the theory determines are basic to all functional human beings:

- breathing
- eating and drinking
- eliminating
- controlling body temperature
- mobilizing
- sleeping
- maintaining a safe environment
- communicating
- personal care and dressing
- working and playing
- expressing sexuality
- dying

Imagine that a man comes into the hospital in congestive heart failure (CHF). Medically, this means that the patient's left ventricle is not working well, causing less blood to be pumped out of the body and a back up of fluid in the venous system, causing congestion in the lungs and extremities. To fix it, you get rid of the fluid and/or improve the function of the left ventricle. Now, the nurse knows the patient has CHF, and she understands the physiology, but to the nurse, the real problem is patient can't breathe like he used to. Since he can't breathe, he can't do all the things he normally does. His life has changed. To help the patient regain normal functioning the nurse not only administers diuretics and medications to strengthen the ventricle, but also assists the patient in doing the things he used to do until such time as he can once again do those things for himself.

Building off nursing theory, about 40 years ago an organization called the North American Nursing Diagnosis Association, or NANDA, created a whole system of assessment called Nursing Diagnoses. A nursing diagnosis is a determination of what the patient's problem is in terms of what the patient's experience of the disease is. NANDA would list the following nursing diagnoses for our patient with CHF:

1. Impaired Gas Exchange related to changes in alveolar capillary membranes.
2. Activity Intolerance related to imbalance between oxygen supply and demand.
3. Altered Peripheral Tissue Perfusion related to decreased blood flow in the peripheral area secondary to decreased cardiac output.
4. Anxiety related to tissue oxygenation disorders, stress due to difficulty in breathing and the knowledge that the heart is not functioning properly.
5. Disturbed Sleep Pattern related to waking up frequently secondary to respiratory disorders.

Does all this nursing theory sound to you like bogus semantics, rhetoric, and academic double-speak? You're not alone. Few practicing nurses use either nursing theories or nursing diagnoses. Most nurses are totally fine with the patient having CHF rather than Activity Intolerance. What these philosophies and models are attempting to do is to define what makes professional nursing different from other healthcare professions. When you ask nurses why they prefer nursing to medicine, it is these underlying philosophies that they are often referring to, consciously or subconsciously.

You kind of need to buy into at least the basic philosophy of nursing if you want to be happy with nursing as your choice. Remember, without nurses there's no patient care, no hospitals, no healing.

Recommended Reading

Black, Beth Perry. *Professional Nursing: concepts and challenges.* 7th ed. Elsevier, Missouri, 2014.

Nightingale, Florence. *Notes on Nursing: What it is, and what it is not.* Dover Books on Biology, 1969.

Nursing Diagnoses 2015-2017, Definitions and Classification. 10th ed. By NANDA International. Wiley Blackwell, New York, 2015.

Roper, nancy, Winifred Logan, Allison Tierney. *The Roper Logan Tierney Model of Nursing.* 5th ed. Churchill Livingstone, 2000.

CHAPTER 5

WHAT DO NURSES DO?

Being a nurse comes with a vast amount of responsibility. Think about it. Why is a person admitted to a hospital? Is it because they need a doctor? No, if he or she needs a doctor the person goes to the doctor's office. If someone is admitted to a hospital it is because that person needs a nurse.

Florence Nightingale herself understood this quite well:

In watching diseases, both in private houses and in public hospitals, the thing which strikes the experienced observer most forcibly is this, that the symptoms or the sufferings generally considered to be inevitable and incident to the disease are very often not symptoms of the disease at all, but of something quite different - of the want of fresh air, or of light, or of warmth, or of quiet, or of cleanliness, or of punctuality and care in the administration of diet, of each or of all of these. And this is true as much in private as in hospital nursing. The reparative process which Nature has instituted and which we call disease, has been hindered by some want of knowledge or attention, in one or in all of these things, and pain, suffering, or interruption of the whole process sets in. If a patient is cold, if a patient is feverish, if a patient is faint, if he is sick after taking food, if he has a bed-sore, it is generally the fault not of the disease, but of the nursing.

Most people think that the job of the nurse is to give patients medications and bedpans and carry out orders. Many consider it a menial job. Nurses do medicate, take care of the physical needs of others, and carry out the plan determined by the care team. There are menial parts of the job, no question. What people don't realize is that the true value of the good nurse lies in his or her ability to *observe and advocate.*

Observing

The nurse is charged with being the first, and sometimes the only, person to notice when something is wrong. The "menial" tasks of physical care take on a new meaning when you realize this. When the nurse cleans a patient's back she is also looking for bedsores. When the nurse helps someone out of a chair he is observing range of motion and strength. When the nurse brings water or food she is looking at how the patient swallows or how nauseous she is, or if the patient has trouble feeding himself. When the nurse brings you pain medication he is observing what your pain level is, if the medication is adequate, and whether the pain is decreasing appropriately or increasing, signaling a problem. When the nurse hands you that paper gown at the doctor's office she is observing your manner, mood, anxiety level, and presence of discomfort. When the nurse takes a patient's vital signs he is observing a patient's skin, noticing he needs a shave or that he hasn't bathed, or that she is having trouble breathing or has been crying. It's hard not to create a human bond with a person while wiping their backside or holding back their hair as they lean over the toilet.

Advocating

One of the biggest misconceptions about nursing is that nurses "just carry out doctor's orders." Well, yes, someone has to do the actual medicating, bandaging, etc. While it is true that the nurse is the one who has to carry out a treatment plan often dictated by someone else, a good nurse advocates for the patient and intervenes when necessary to ensure the correct care is given. Any good nurse knows that in July, when newly minted doctors arrive to inflict their inexperience on everyone, she'd better check and re-check those medication orders for accuracy. If a patient is in pain and has not been ordered adequate pain medication, the nurse's job is to page and call and push until he gets the appropriate pain medication orders. The nurse explains things to a confused patient and family. A grieving mother of a stillborn can be found a room on a non-maternity floor so she doesn't have to hear the cries of babies. The nurse makes that happen. Maybe a patient who is dying wants to see his dog before he dies. The nurse can make that happen.

Teamwork

The most common task of most interns is to "write orders", i.e, to list what must be done for a patient in terms of meds, diet, activity, etc. I actually hate the word "order" when talking about what has been prescribed for a patient. It is sort of militaristic and it reinforces the hierarchical structure in hospitals that is so often unhelpful. I would prefer something like "Hey, would you help me and the patient out here by doing what we've all decided together is best for the patient. I can't do it myself, I need your help." Because that's what *should* be happening.

Here is where I have to address one of the fundamental frustrations of nursing, and it is very important that you understand this. In many settings, nurses have *a great deal of responsibility and not a lot of power.* Decisions are made without nursing input. Calls for medications are forgotten or ignored. Dietary preferences are communicated and not considered. Orders spit out of computers without the nurse being informed that the orders have been written. Hours go by after an urgent call made by a nurse about a suspicious-looking wound. In a good working environment doctors and nurses work together as teams, with mutual respect and clear communication channels, in which treatment plans are decided upon as a group and the plan is carried out collaboratively. This does not always happen.

Practicalities

The day-to-day life of a nurse is not easy. It is not a desk job. There is a lot of physical labor. Your feet hurt. Your back hurts. You spend too much time on the computer. Patients are demanding. Doctors are demanding. You ride herd on surgeons who don't complete their pre-op paperwork and interns who forget to write diet orders. You realize you're the only person who knows that the test that was just ordered requires that the patient not eat for 8 hours or that that scan requires intravenous access. People cry on you and poop on you. There are a lot of rules. Not everyone is nice to you.

In order to be happy in nursing, you have to embrace, or at least at some deep level be on board with, the philosophies of nursing described in the previous chapter. You have to find the joy in a nicely dressed wound or a newly clean bed, because you know you are watching over your patient and advocating for their right to surroundings that are optimal for healing.

CHAPTER 6

NURSING EDUCATION

One of the strengths of nursing as a profession is that there are a number of ways to get in. This is also one of nursing's weaknesses, as we will see in a later chapter.

Associate's Degree in Nursing (ADN)

Before World War II most nurses were educated in 3-year, hospital-based nursing schools. The quality of these programs varied widely. Doctors who owned hospitals would open nursing schools to ensure a steady stream of cheap labor. Hospital nursing supervisors were often also the nursing school head and its primary nursing instructor. Nurses were taught about whatever illnesses were usually treated at the specific hospital in which they trained. Nurses did not have college degrees.

During WWII the shortage of nurses created a need for shorter, 2-year training programs, which eventually migrated to community colleges. Registration for nurses followed with the development of nurse's associations and regulatory legislation. The ADN is a remnant of this history. You can become a Registered Nurse (RN) in this country with just this 2-year degree.

Here's what you have to do:
1. Have a high school diploma or GED
2. Have a high school GPA of at least 2.5
3. Have passed high school chemistry and biology with a C or better (or do these classes as part of the degree program)
4. Be competent in math with a 25 on the SAT or an ACT of 18
5. Have a negative drug screen and criminal background check
6. Keep a 2.0 GPA in your ADN program
7. Have at least a C in all your courses and a B- in the nursing classes

Here are the nursing courses you might take in an ADN program (my thanks to Grand Rapids Community College):

• Perspectives in Nursing
• Application of Basic Nursing Skills
• Nursing Practice Concepts 1 and 2
• Health Illness Concepts 1-4
• Population Health
• Anatomy and Physiology
• Biology

Bachelor of Science in Nursing (BSN)

As professional groups and employers pushed for more education and as studies came out linking better patient care to better-educated nurses, colleges started offering Bachelor's degrees in nursing. BSN training combines the practical skills of the ADN with more theory, public health education, and research. You generally get a more extensive liberal arts education than an ADN program would provide. BSN programs typically require that you have a high school GPA of around 3 and higher standardized test scores, with SATs in the 900s. These are general minimum requirements, although specific schools may have higher standards. Here is what one of my blog readers said:

Yes, you have to have a decent GPA in high school. BUT. You also have to have taken ALL of the prerequisites and gotten at least a B. This includes college algebra, college biology, the entire year of anatomy and physiology, microbiology, psychology, english 101 and 102, and a sociology class. GPAs are taken into consideration along with HESI test scores, and I'm pretty sure someone with a 75 wouldn't even be considered for a nursing program here. Competition is TOUGH. Most of the people I know that are currently in nursing school had 4.0 GPAs before getting in.

(The HESI this writer is referring to is Health Education Systems Incorporated, a company that provides exams and other study material to help prepare student nurses for their professional licensure exam. Schools often use HESI to help predict the students likelihood of success in licensing exams. Their Admission Assessment Exams are used as a baseline entrance criterion by some nursing schools.)

RN to BSN Programs

Many schools now offer an ADN to RN option, in which the training and classwork of the ADN curriculum is expanded and the the requirements for a college degree are added. These very popular programs are good options for people who need to work while getting their degree.

Non-nurse College Graduate Programs

This sort of program is what I did. It allows people who have college degrees in some other area of life to obtain the coursework they need to be eligible to sit for the RN exam, called the NCLEX. These programs, sometimes called accelerated nursing programs, come in two forms. Accelerated baccalaureate programs take a year or two and generally don't result in an additional degree. The other program structure takes three years to complete and results in a master's degree. The three-year program usually allows you to take the NCLEX after the 2nd year.

For the purposes of this book it is very important to understand what I am about to say.

None of the above classwork transfers to medical school. Even the BSN won't help you unless you've taken the full battery of pre-med classes. Everyone in medical school starts from the beginning.

CHAPTER 7

WHAT IS MEDICINE?

Medicine, of course, has been around forever. From the "four humors" theory of the 16th century to the discovery of antibiotics in the 1900s to robotic surgery today, medicine has changed drastically and continues to do so. One thing that hasn't changed is this: medicine is the diagnosis and treatment of *disease.*

The Medical Model

The focus of medicine on the disease process is one of the main things that distinguishes medical education from nursing education. The focus is not, or hasn't traditionally been, on the treatment of the patient but the treatment of the disease. This concept is the basis of the Medical Model. It looks like this:

1. Complaint: Patient comes in with a symptom
2. History and physical examination: The doctor talks to the patient and examines him or her to create a list of possible disease processes that could be going on inside the patient
3. Ancillary tests: The doctor does various tests to determine which of the possible diseases is most likely given the data.
4. Diagnosis: The doctor decides what is wrong.
5. Treatment: The doctor decides what to do.

To illustrate how this works, let's take our congestive heart failure example from chapter 4. If you remember, the nursing model of congestive heart failure says that the problem is that the patient is having trouble living his life as he is accustomed to because of symptoms of the disease. The job of the nurse is to return the patient to full functioning. In the medical model the problem is that the patient's left ventricle doesn't work. It is the doctor's job to fix the ventricle.

This is what medical school teaches you. If you want to diagnose and treat disease, you have to go to medical school. No place does it better. Medical school courses are designed to give the student knowledge of medicine. It is not, especially in the first two years, designed to teach students anything at all about taking care of people. The only thing medical students are qualified for when they graduate is more training. An MD without a residency qualifies you for nothing, at least nothing in clinical practice.

The Human Element

The above is not to say that doctors are all heartless automatons doling out bad news and dangerous drugs. Recent trends in medical training have sought to shift some emphasis onto the human interaction between patient and doctor. Through longitudinal patient experiences, classes, arts, journaling, and outreach programs to underserved neighborhoods, medical schools are acknowledging the need for empathetic and caring physicians.

The truth is that most medical students go into medical school because they really want to take care of people. It's the training process that decreases that empathetic instinct. The difficulties of residency decrease young doctors' ability to see past their own suffering to the suffering of others. Mature physicians tend to gain that human element back.

Most doctors are kind, caring, and want what's best for the patient both medically and holistically. They just come at it from a different angle.

CHAPTER 8

MEDICAL EDUCATION

It is no secret that getting into medical school can be difficult. The academic bar is set high. It wasn't always thus. In the 1800s a man (it was always a man) could become a doctor simply by apprenticing with another doctor. Before that doctors didn't really have any specific training at all. Over time, medical school evolved from apprenticeships to informal two-year programs of study to four-year clinical training without residency to the formal undergraduate - medical school - residency - fellowship slog that we have today.

Historically, becoming a physician didn't necessarily require high achievement in the undergraduate years. Admission to medical school had more to do with social position and wealth. Some would say it still does. The system has evolved to favor those who excel academically, and in another book we can discuss the societal and economic pressures that promote or discourage such achievement.

Pre-med

There is no such thing as a Bachelor of Pre-med. You can get into medical school with any undergraduate degree, as long as you fulfill the admissions requirements. You can be an English major and still get into medical school as long as you also do all the science and math. The reasons pre-med is so heavy on math and science have to do with both the subject matter of medicine and the discipline required to get through the education process. Much of medicine is science-based, of course, so a good understanding of things like biology are useful. On the other hand, I don't remember anything about physics, calculus, or organic chemistry, but taking, and doing well in, those classes taught me the mental discipline, problem-solving skills, and determination that medical school required. Pre-med requirements are typically as follows:

1.1 year of biology
2.1 year of chemistry with lab
3.1 year of organic chemistry with lab
4.1 year of physics with lab (with or without calculus)
5.1-2 semesters of calculus

These must be full basic science classes. "Chemistry for Nurses" or "Intro to Biology" won't cut it. And you must do well in these classes. You don't have to go to a fancy school, although it helps. You just have to study hard.

I reiterate. You could have three PhDs and regularly report to Congress and the Pope but you won't get into medical school if you don't have these courses. If you don't have them, you have to go get them. Community colleges often have them. Some medical schools sponsor post-baccalaureate pre-med programs (a "post-bac") These programs will often save a place for the post-bac student in the medical school contingent on the student's performance in classes and on the MCAT.

The MCAT

MCAT stands for Medical College Admissions Test. Most medical schools require this standardized test. I'm not going to say much about it here. If you are not a science-y type of person (like me), this test will probably be hard for you. Some people spend hundreds of dollars for test prep, some take it cold.

Medical School

All med schools teach the same thing more or less, though the method of instruction can be different. The first two years are sort of like drinking from a firehose. The second two are classically called "the clinical years". You can't cut it shorter than 4 years, but the good news is that it is very difficult to flunk out of medical school. After all the work you did to stay on top of your class in the pre-med courses, the traditional pass/fail system in most medical schools feels like a relief.

Classically, courses in the first two years center around anatomy, physiology, and pathophysiology, although the style and format of the classes varies widely among medical schools. Some go with the straight lecture-test model. Others use a more small-group, trial-and-error arrangement, like collaborative creation of decision trees, flow charts, and discussion groups. Most use a combination of educational techniques. New students often ask - how much of this do I really need to know for the test? The answer is: all of it. Prepare to memorize. How much of it will the student remember? Depends. A student who goes into orthopedics will remember a lot more about bones than your average nephrologist. The point of the first two years is to provide students a solid grounding in the science of medicine, which is the whole point of medical school and part of what makes it unique training.

The second two years focus more on clinical training, putting the science into practice. Many medical schools actually include clinical experiences in the first two years as well, typically in the primary care setting. The quality and value of the experiences you get in the clinical years will vary widely, depending on your own interest, the quality of the teachers, the involvement (or non-involvement) of the residents, the type of setting, attitudes of the staff towards students, and a million other factors. The most successful students in these years are those who observe carefully and respectfully, act enthusiastic, and keep their mouths shut. You will not learn how to be a doctor in the clinical years. You will learn a whole lot about how the system works.

It is important to understand that the kinds of experiences you have in the clinical years of medical school can and will color your impressions of each specialty, so be careful. You might hate obstetrics because the residents treated you terribly, wouldn't let you deliver any babies, and made you do the night shift 8 days in a row. Even if you were interested in OB to begin with. You might love cardiology because you had a great mentor and published a scientific paper on valve disease. Even if you planned to be a surgeon. The trick is to separate the personalities from the work itself.

The Match

The clinical years are also when you have to decide what kind of medicine you would like to pursue. This is because during the end of the third year and all of the fourth year many students are consumed with landing a good residency in their chosen field. This involves traveling for interviews, evaluating programs, sensing how the various residencies treat their residents, how rigorous the training is, etc. After completing this process, you submit a list of your choices, ranked first to last. All the residency programs to which you've applied then submit *their* rank lists. These lists are shaken up in a computer program and, on "Match Day", everyone gets an envelope indicating where they will be going for residency. That's it. That's where you go. No negotiation. Got a residency in Boston but have a significant other in California? Too bad. Got kids in school in Atlanta but got matched in Dallas? Too bad.

Residency

Here is where you really learn how to be a doctor. No other training is as thorough as residency. Nobody else in the business has done more clinical training hours than the doctor. It is long, and it is hard.

CHAPTER 9

ADVANCED PRACTICE NURSING

Many people ask me about choosing a "mid-level" degree such as nurse practitioner or physician's assistant. These are great options and a lot of happy people go this route. Be careful that you understand how these roles fit in, or don't fit in, to the health care scene today. The American Association of Colleges of Nursing (AACN) defines advanced nursing practice as "Any form of nursing intervention that influences health care outcomes for individuals or populations, including the direct care of individual patients, management of care for individuals and populations, administration of nursing and health care organizations, and the development and implementation of health policy." Not a terribly helpful definition. Here are some of the certifications that come under the umbrella of advanced practice nursing (APN):

Certified Nurse Midwife

The CNM certification evolved from the historical role of the midwife. Many CNMs work happily alongside obstetricians at hospitals around the country.

Certified Registered Nurse Anesthetist

The CRNA has developed over time in the same way that anesthesia has. The earliest experts in anesthesia were actually nurses trained to do the work that had been farmed out to the most junior intern or medical student. Surgeons were understandably happier with the services of these women (they were all women) than they were with the inexperienced students. This unusual nursing function allowed early regulatory efforts by nurse associations, which is why the CRNA role has evolved in a consistent and defined manner.

Clinical Nurse Specialist

CNSs became popular in the 1950s and 60s, coinciding with the evolution of nursing theory. The focus is on consultation, research, staff education, patient/family education, care coordination, and institutional management. The CNS role has more recently been deemed as too expensive by hospital administrators, both because of the CNS indirect role in patient care and their lack of clearly defined and consistent responsibilities. Each CNS makes her own way and develops, and defends, her own role. You will still find CNSs in community and long-term care settings as patients are discharged earlier from acute care hospitals and chronic care becomes increasingly complicated.

Nurse Practitioner

In the 1960s federal legislation expanded Medicare and Medicaid services in the US. This created a shortage of primary care medical providers, especially in poor and underserved areas. The earliest concept in the minds of both doctors and nurses was that the NP role was a way for doctors to extend care for their patients. The first nurse practitioner program was actually created by a nurse and a physician working together. As such, the role first developed outside of nursing education in continuing education programs and were collaborative efforts between medicine and nursing. NPs are especially helpful in areas of primary care, health promotion and community/public health, although today you find them in all areas of health care.

Physician's Assistant

PAs are not nurses. They are educated and certified outside of nursing. I include them here because they have many of the same roles that NPs do. According to the Yale School of Medicine, which itself has a PA program, the education of PAs first started around 1965 in response to the same shortage and maldistribution of physicians that fueled the rise of NPs. Just like NPs, PAs were trained to provide medical care to rural and underserved populations but, unlike NPs, many PAs do not have graduate degrees, although the Association of Physician Assistant Programs has recommended that the PA certification should move in that direction. It is important to note that PAs are educated in the medical model and are specifically defined as "a health professional who practices medicine with the supervision of a licensed physician" (American Academy of Physician Assistants).

In my experience PAs today work in hospitals assisting surgeons and providing support services in the areas of post-op care, admissions, orders, and follow-up. A word of warning here - I am not a PA and my direct experience with PAs is limited. I encourage the reader to find some PAs and ask them about what their roles are and the educational path they took. In later editions I will expand on this section.

ADVANCED PRACTICE NURSING EDUCATION

Virtually all NPs, CNMs, CNSs and CRNAs have graduate degrees. These degrees can be subsequent to a traditional BSN, or there are programs for college graduates with non-nursing degrees who want to transition to nursing. The training is usually 2-3 years. APN education expands the fund of knowledge in a number of ways. Students are trained in research methods and statistics, population and global health, and have additional training in physiology and pathophysiology. None of these courses, by the way, can be transferred to medical school. While there is more focus on diagnosis and treatment, the milieu of APN programs remains firmly in nursing philosophy. Happy nurse practitioners are not doctors and do not wish they were.

Where APN education differs perhaps most significantly from traditional nursing education is in the clinical realm. Most NP programs require upwards of 600 hours of clinical practice under the guidance of an NP, an MD, or PA, usually in primary care practice. These hours are divided into acute outpatient facilities like walk-in clinics as well as in-hospital work and primary care offices. The emphasis is on primary, outpatient, ambulatory care.

Not all APN programs require a traditional academic master's thesis. Some have final projects involving community medicine, outreach, or education. These programs focus most on the clinical aspect of advanced practice nursing. Those programs that do require a thesis tend to be the more research-focused programs that view the role of the NP in a more academic sense. It is important when choosing a program to know which kind of focus you are looking for. Nursing research tends to be more clinically focused than work done by physicians, but it doesn't have to be. A nurse with a solid background in science who wants to do basic lab research can certainly do so. The range of subjects you can address is wide, from hard statistical analysis to "soft" science topics like patient perspective or stress management.

The Nursing Doctorate

Nursing has awarded doctorates for many years. These used to be mostly PhD or a Doctor of Nursing Science (DNSc) degrees and are primarily research degrees designed to train educators. Some nursing leaders have advocated introducing a new clinical doctorate, the Doctor of Nursing pPractice or DNP. No one is quite sure yet what it would entail. The AACN has come up with some curricular recommendations.

1. Scientific underpinnings for practice
2. Organizational and system leadership for quality improvement and systems thinking
3. Clinical scholarship and analytical methods for evidence-based practice
4. Information systems/technology and patient care technology for the improvement and transformation of health care
5. Health care policy for advocacy in health care
6. Inter-professional collaboration for improving patient and population health outcomes
7. Clinical prevention and population health for improving the nation's health
8. Advanced nursing practice

What does all that mean? Do these eight points help you understand why you might want to be a DNP? Not really. DNP programs are supposed to be the ultimate nursing clinical degree. DNPs receive 1000 hours of clinical practicum instead of 600, and in place of a dissertation many do final projects like practice change initiatives. It remains to be seen whether DNP programs grow in favor as a preferred preparatory path for nurse practitioners, or if the degree becomes more of an access point for nursing leadership and policy rather than actual clinical care.

CHAPTER 10

POLICY AND POLITICS IN NURSING

Why do nurses need to care about policy and politics? Policy determines each and every thing the APRN, or any health professional, can do, and just as important, whether or not he or she will get paid for their services. Here's Dr. Margaret Moss:

I think you need to know policy because policy touches everything you do. It is guiding who you can see, when you can see them, how often you can see them, how much you are going to get paid for seeing them, where you can see them, everything.

There are a few things about nursing that make the politics tricky. I discuss a few of them here but be aware that there are competing views on either side of the proverbial aisle on all these issues.

Image

Nursing has sometimes been accused of having an image problem that medicine doesn't have. This difficulty stems from a number of factors, not all of which have to do with nursing itself. The journal Advanced Critical Care Nursing published an article in 2004 in which the authors observe that:

When asked to put a mental picture to the word "nurse", the image people see is often far removed from the image nurses wish to project. Many see nurses as handmaidens to physicians, wearing white caps and stockings, and surrendering their chairs to physicians. Others see unflattering images from the media. Nursing's tarnished image is partially responsible for the perception of oppression in nursing. Much of nursing's image problem relates to how nurses perceive and use power.

Here are some of the factors influencing both the image nurses project and the image they take upon themselves.

1. <u>Nursing is still a predominantly female profession.</u>

The US Department of Health and Human Services reports that in 2010 only 6.6% of nurses were male and only 16.8% were non-white or hispanic. Combine these facts with the gender inequity in pay, cultural norms around female leadership and family roles, and the under-representation of girls in STEM classes, and you come up with the lack of respect inherent in a "woman's career".

Medicine, while 50% female in medicals schools, is still very much a man's world. Women who want to succeed in medicine must still conform to the demands of a field that assumes someone else is tending to the home fires.

2. <u>Nursing still does not require a college degree.</u>

The existence of an entry point into nursing that does not require a 4-year degree fuels the impression of nurses as unintelligent or as "handmaids of physicians". While ADNS are great nurses, nursing policy makers would really like to make a college degree a requirement for RN licensure. The American Nurses Association (ANA) Board of Directors in 2000 reaffirmed its longstanding position that baccalaureate education should be the standard for entry into professional nursing. There is disagreement about this among nursing educators. Some argue that any barrier to entry could discourage students from going into nursing.

Medicine, by contrast, has an incredibly high barrier to entry. The profession seems to discourage young people from going into medicine on purpose. To become a doctor you have to perform at a very high level for a very long time from a relatively young age, and there are no shortcuts. For better or worse, this reality gives doctors an image of superiority that they may or may not deserve.

3. Stereotypes are easy to perpetuate.

The images of nursing in popular culture also contribute to nursing's image problem. Consider Nurse Ratchett from *One Flew Over the Cuckoo's Nest;* Dixie, the only nurse in the whole of "Emergency!"'s hospital; Hot Lips Houlihan in the 1970s show M*A*S*H; those comic books depicting the nurse with the big breasts and short skirts; and most recently the drug-addicted Nurse Jackie.

3. Nurses are largely absent in health policy debates.

Nursing is not well-represented at the health policy table, although its presence is increasing. Here's a story Margaret Moss tells about her experiences in Washington, DC when she was a fellow at the Robert Wood Johnson Foundation:

I go to DC. I'm the only nurse in my cohort, the seven of us from the Robert Wood Johnson Fellowship. As we arrived we were wooed by the AMA, the AAMC, and so forth. They're taking us out to lunch, they're inviting us to wingdings, they're having one on one meetings with each of us. What did I get from the ANA? I got a one paragraph letter: "Dear Margaret, we're so proud of you, we're here if you need us and good luck". Come on. Nursing needs to step up, big time. There are three million nurses in the US, and yet it's pretty silent out there."

In politics, money often speaks louder than words. In 2008 the ANA gave $562,000 to federal candidates through its political action group. The total amount of professional association contributions from the healthcare sector overall was in excess of $95,000,000.

Scope of Practice

The APN role has evolved and diversified over the years. Most APN-physician working relationships are uniquely defined depending on the needs of the practice and the skill set of each party. This collaboration almost always creates a happy work environment for everyone. In clinical practice, on an individual level, APNs and physicians work in harmony. At the policy level however, not so much.

With the increased role of NPs in primary care, and as hospital administrators have seen an advantage in this lower-cost group, arguments about turf, especially within the primary care community, have been escalating. Nurses have been pushing for greater independence of practice and doctors are saying that, in essence, nurses are not doctors and should not act as such. At issue is the definition of "full scope of practice."

In 2010 the Institute of Medicine (IOM), a non-profit under the umbrella of the National Academy of Sciences that takes evidence-based recommendation for public health and science policy, teamed up with the Robert Wood Johnson Foundation, the nations largest public health philanthropy, to develop a series of recommendations called *The Future of Nursing: Leading Change, Advancing Health*. Here are the four key messages:

1. Nurses should practice to the full extent of their education and training.
2. Nurses should achieve higher levels of education and training through an improved education system that promotes seamless academic progression.
3. Nurses should be full partners, with physicians and other health care professionals, in redesigning health care in the United States.
4. Effective workforce planning and policy making require better data collection and information infrastructure.

It is the first message that has the policy wonks in both medicine and nursing in a tizzy. What exactly is practicing to the full extent of education and training? Depends whom you ask. Doctors say APRNs should only practice under the supervision of doctors, and nurses say they shouldn't need such supervision. Each side uses economic and safety arguments to boost their cases, and both medicine and nursing have spent a lot of money on scholarly studies trying to prove that the other side is less safe or cost more. Committees have been set up. Projects have been planned and associations have been formed.

Why should we care? All of us in the trenches are just going to keep working together anyway, right? All this controversy could have remained isolated in the halls of national and state legislative bodies except that it hasn't. Patients see the fighting and get confused. Who should I see for my upper respiratory infection? Can I trust what my NP says? Should I insist that a doctor treat my kid's sore throat? Everybody wears a white coat, how can I tell the difference?

It is important to care because people will ask.

The Knowledge Debate

One of the main arguments the medical professions have to the practice of NPs is that APRNs "don't have enough knowledge." This is true; APRNs don't have as much *medical* knowledge, and their clinical training hours are not as numerous as those you would acquire in a medical residency. The question is, do you need the high level of training acquired in medical school in all patient encounters, of all types, in all settings?

I'm a violinist, so I'm going to use music as a way to illustrate how I look at the knowledge debate. When a violinist practices (clinical training) over time she is exposed to every technical difficulty (disease) she could possibly encounter, repeatedly, in multiple settings. The goal of practice is to recognize the difficulty (diagnosis) and figure out ways to overcome it (treatment).

Now, a violinist who has been practicing for, say, five years, probably has a solid experience of the basics of violin playing (clinical training). She has not encountered every difficulty (disease) out there but is fairly confident she can identify basic problems (diagnosis) and come up with solutions (treatment). She is qualified to confidently play pieces of music within her experience base. She is not going to go play the Tchaikovsky Violin Concerto or audition for the New York Philharmonic. She is not qualified to do so and wouldn't want to. This does not make her a less intelligent or less gifted violinist than a more advanced player. If she wants to play for the New York Philharmonic, she will have to devote more years of practice and specialized training to become qualified for the more complex work that job requires.

The APRN has clinical training (practice) that qualifies her to diagnose and treat basic problems. This does not make her less intelligent or less gifted than the doctor. She does not address complex medical issues (i.e, the NY Phil or heart surgery) and doesn't want to. If she does want to, she has to go to medical school.

Recommended reading:

DeNisco, S and Barker, A, Eds. *Advanced Practice Nursing: Evolving Roles for the Transformation of the Profession.* 2nd ed. Jones and Bartlett Learning, Burlington, MA, 2013.

Hain, D and Fleck, L. *Barriers to NP practice that impact healthcare redesign.* OJIN, 19(2), May 2014.

Inglehart, John. *Expanding the role of advanced nurse practitioners - risks and rewards.* N Engl J Med 368(20), May 2013.

Milstead, Jeri, Ed. *Health Policy and Politics, a nurse's guide.* 4th ed. Jones and Bartlett learning, Burlington, MA, 2013.

CHAPTER 11

THOUGHTS ON BRAINS, MONEY, YOUTH, AND LIFESTYLE
(Or, The Opinion Page)

Let's talk about elephants!

When I was writing this little book I had an interesting response from some of the people I told about it. "Wait," they would say, "is the nursing vs. medicine question even a thing? People who become nurses aren't capable of being doctors because they either don't have the smarts, don't have the money, or... ." and here they trail off because what they are really suggesting is that nurses and doctors are separated by *class distinction*. This is what we might call the proverbial elephant in the room.

It is true that, in the US, the people who become doctors tend to come from wealthier families than nurses, they tend to have family members who are physicians, and they certainly have educational advantages that they may or may not have taken advantage of. The number one reason for this is that, in the US, medical school is not free. In Sweden, Finland, and Norway, it is free. In many EU countries undergraduate school and medical school is combined into 6 years for a fraction of the cost. The average medical school in the the US costs between $200,000 and $325,000, according to the American Association of Medical Colleges. There are loans, grants, and loan-forgiveness programs such as the National Health Service Corps, and the military will pay for school if you give them back a certain number of years. All of this aid, however, is contingent on the student having large swaths of years to spend repaying debt, either by time or by money, while making relatively little. Medical school is not flexible, and does not make allowances for students who really need to support themselves. So it is certainly easier to become a doctor if you have money.

I had no money. My mom is a music teacher and my dad a minister. I'm paying $1000 per month for 30 years to pay back my debts. In the world I grew up in, such expensive education was unthinkable. But I have the advantage of parents who value education and believe you can go after the things you want. Not everyone has that advantage. For people like me, we can only go to medical school (or nursing school actually) if we think we can, if someone in our lives encourages us and motivates us, if we know where to reach out for funding and advice, and if we really, really want it. For many this is true of nursing school as well, especially 4-year programs.

All this does not mean that people of reduced circumstances are not *capable* of becoming doctors or bachelor-prepared nurses. Nor does it mean that being a doctor or BSN makes you a superior individual. **None of this has anything to do with smarts or ability or talent or character**. Higher education doesn't take brains so much as it takes persistence and a whole lot of support. Some people are born with built-in supports. Others have to make their own.

Let's talk (more) about money!

The Bureau of Labor Statistics, a division of the US Department of Labor tells us that the average physician salary is in the range of $200,000 per year. This number varies widely depending on what kind of medicine you practice and where, but still, it is a pretty good number. Let's break that number down a bit.

Let's say the average guy coming out of college can get a job that pays $40,000 per year. Medical school and residency lasts about 8 years on average. Residency pays around $50,000 per year (about $10.00 per hour!) So your college friends are already $120,000 in earnings ahead of you. The average debt of students graduating from medical school is around $170,000. Paid over 30 years the cost of that loan is maybe $425,000. This means that your average doctor finishes training about $550,000 in the hole. With no savings, no retirement.

Then you get your first job, and suddenly you're rich! $200,000 per year breaks down to $16,666 per month or $3846 per week. But you don't get all 200K of course. You get more like $128,000 after taxes, which breaks down to $10,600 per month. The cost of rent is, say, $1000/month. Your student loan puts you back another $1000 per month or so. That new car you just bought is another $300 plus utilities, car insurance, gas, food... I'll estimate your monthly expenses around $3,600 (to make the math easy). You still have $7000 per month free and clear. Except you won't live forever, so there's retirement to think about, and you're already 8 years behind in saving for retirement. Plus, you want to own a home someday so you have to save for the down payment on that. Also, you want to have a child as soon as possible because the clock is ticking after all, and a nanny (which you will need of course given your schedule) will run you another $3,000 per month. Then there's saving for college...

You see my point. While doctors aren't starving, they're not buying Lear jets either. In my neighborhood the people with the big houses on 5 acres aren't doctors. They're NFL players. You will be comfortable, but you won't be rich.

Meanwhile, the nurse working with you is making around $75,000 per year. $75,000 is, incidentally, the inflection point for money buying happiness. It's generally understood that people get happier the more they make up until $75,000 and then the curve drops off. That's $54,000 after taxes, or $4,440 per month. S/he has student loan debt, too, as much as any average college graduate, about $30,000. The nurse is not, however, in the hole for all those lost wages. He got a job right out of college and started saving for retirement right away. She decided to have a child but has a very flexible schedule and doesn't need a nanny (unless she wants one of course). The nurse practitioner down the street has more debt and more lost wages but also makes about $100,000 on average, meaning that generally speaking s/he sort of balances out right about where the RN does.

All this is to say that money is a very poor reason to choose any field in health care. You want to make money? Invent something everyone wants or go invest other people's money.

Let's talk about age!

The saying goes "You're never too old to…" do whatever it is the person you're saying this to wants to do. The fact is that, no, you might not be too old, but you probably are encumbered by accumulated life in the form of children, spouses, home ownership, aging parents, the need to make a living, etc. You can do anything you want. More life just makes it a little more difficult.

Let's talk about having it all!

So many people ask me questions that relate to work-life balance. Here's how Wikipedia, that repository of all wisdom, defines work-life balance: *Work–life balance is a concept including the proper prioritization between work (career and ambition) and lifestyle (health, pleasure, leisure, family).*

Notice that this definition separates career from pleasure. In an ideal world, we would all get paid to do things that give us pleasure. In the real world, most of us do work to make a living so we can go do something we really like after work. If you have to work so much doing something that gives you no pleasure that you never have time to do anything that gives you pleasure, well, you have a work-life balance problem. This imbalance is felt across industries. Nursing journals have just as many articles about lifestyle and stress as medical journals do. Nurses burn out just as often as doctors do. A nurse who is working nights one week and days the next week is no more capable of taking care of himself and his family than the doctor who's on call every third night.

No one has work-life balance. Everyone juggles. Choose what work you want to do based on what gives you pleasure, not based on how much time off you get. Life is what's going on while you're doing stuff. A good life is what's going on while you're doing stuff you like.

Made in the USA
San Bernardino, CA
13 May 2020